COMPACT GUIDES TO FITNESS & HEALTH

LIVING DISEASE-FREE:
STRATEGIES FOR REDUCING YOUR RISK OF DISEASE

CONTENT PROVIDED BY MAYO CLINIC HEALTH INFORMATION

MASON CREST PUBLISHERS
Philadelphia, Pennsylvania

Living Disease-Free: Strategies for Reducing Your Risk of Disease provides reliable, practical information on adopting healthy habits to remain in sound health. Much of the information comes directly from the experience of Mayo Clinic physicians, nurses, registered dietitians, health educators and other health care professionals. This book supplements the advice of your personal physician, whom you should consult for individual medical problems. MAYO, MAYO CLINIC, MAYO CLINIC HEALTH INFORMATION and the Mayo triple-shield logo are marks of Mayo Foundation for Medical Education and Research.

Hardcover Library Edition Published 2002
Mason Crest Publishers
370 Reed Road
Suite 302
Broomall, PA 19008-0914
(866) MCP-BOOK (toll free)

First Printing
1 2 3 4 5 6 7 8 9 10
Library of Congress Cataloging-in-Publication Data on file at the Library of Congress

ISBN 1-59084-257-X (hc)
Printed in the United States of America

Contents

Introduction

Research suggests that your health in later life depends more on your lifestyle choices than your genes. The sooner you adopt healthy habits, the greater your chances of living to a ripe old age. However, you're never too old to start taking steps toward living a longer, healthier life.

This booklet identifies risk factors for these common diseases:

- Heart disease and stroke
- Cancer
- Lung disease
- Diabetes
- Kidney disease

Some risk factors you can't control — but many you can. Learn what you can do right now to help reduce your risk of disease. This booklet will help you take charge of your health and change behaviors that put your health — and ultimately, your life — at risk.

Include your doctor in your plan to improve your health and longevity. Start by scheduling regular medical checkups. These help your doctor assess your overall health as well as your risk factors for disease. In addition, your doctor may recommend specific screening tests based on your age, medical history and lifestyle habits. These help catch potential health problems early — when the odds for successful treatment are greatest.

Assess your risk of disease

Whether you're likely to develop a particular disease depends on your risk factors. A risk factor is anything that makes you susceptible to developing a disease. Some risk factors, such as lifestyle habits, you can control. Other risk factors, such as heredity and sex, you can't. However, it's important to be aware of risk factors you can't control, so you can take appropriate action — scheduling screening tests and trying to reduce your risk by addressing risk factors you can control.

What are your risk factors? Let's look at the risk factors for these common diseases:

- Heart disease and stroke (page 5)
- Cancer (page 9)
- Lung disease (page 13)
- Diabetes (page 15)
- Kidney disease (page 16)

These diseases are featured not only because of their prevalence but also because they have preventable causes. In addition to a list of general risk factors for each disease, you'll find a checklist that helps you identify your own risk factors. Discuss your risk factors with your doctor.

Heart disease and stroke

Nearly a million people die from heart disease and stroke each year in the United States. Heart disease is a general term used to describe many different forms of heart problems. These include coronary artery disease (blockage in the coronary arteries), cardiomyopathy (disease of the heart muscle), heart valve defects, and arrhythmia (irregular heartbeat).

The American Heart Association has identified these risk factors for heart disease:

Risk factors you can control

• **Smoking** — If you smoke, your risk of a heart attack and stroke is twice that of a nonsmoker. Frequent exposure to second-hand smoke puts you at greater risk of heart disease — even if you don't smoke yourself. Bottom line: If you smoke, stop. (For information on how you can stop smoking, see the Stop Smoking Planner on page 29.)

• **High cholesterol** — If you have undesirable cholesterol levels (see chart below), you're more likely to develop heart disease. Your risk is even greater if you also have high blood pressure and smoke. You can lower your cholesterol levels by eating well, exercising regularly and, if necessary, taking medication. Check your cholesterol every 5 years, if your levels are within normal ranges — more frequently if your levels are undesirable.

UNDERSTANDING YOUR CHOLESTEROL LEVELS

	DESIRABLE	BORDERLINE	UNDESIRABLE
Total cholesterol	Below 200	200-239	240 and above
LDL cholesterol	Below 130	130-159	160 and above
HDL cholesterol	Above 45	40-45	Below 40
Triglycerides	Below 150	150-199	200 and above

Levels are in milligrams of cholesterol per deciliter (mg/dL) of blood and apply to adults age 20 and older. Desirable ranges may vary depending on individual health conditions. Check with your doctor.

• **High blood pressure** — If you have high blood pressure, your heart works harder — causing it to enlarge and eventually weaken. High blood pressure increases your risk of having a stroke, heart attack and congestive heart failure. Your risk is even greater if you also are obese, smoke, or have high cholesterol or diabetes.

Your blood pressure tends to increase as you age. Until age 55, men have a greater risk of high blood pressure than women. Between 55 and 75, the risk is about the same for both sexes. After 75, women are more likely than men to develop high blood pressure.

Bottom line: Most people don't even know they have high blood pressure. The condition has few, if any, reliable symptoms. Check your blood pressure at least every 2 years. You can lower your blood pressure by controlling your weight, exercising regularly, eating well, stopping smoking, limiting your use of caffeine and alcohol and, if necessary, taking medication.

UNDERSTANDING YOUR BLOOD PRESSURE MEASUREMENT

	SYSTOLIC		DIASTOLIC
Optimal	Below 120	and	Below 80
Normal	Below 130	and	Below 85
High normal	130-139	or	85-89
*High blood pressure	140 or above	or	90 or above

*Based on the average of two or more readings taken at each of two or more visits after a baseline measurement.

• **Sedentary lifestyle** — Regular exercise helps control cholesterol, diabetes and obesity — all risk factors of heart disease. Regular exercise is important because it increases your heart's ability to pump blood, increases the size of your coronary arteries and reduces the buildup of cholesterol-containing fatty deposits in your blood vessels (atherosclerosis). Exercise also lowers your cholesterol levels and blood pressure. Aim for 3 to 4 hours a week of moderately intense physical activity — such as brisk walking, swimming and biking.

• **Obesity** — You're obese if your body mass index is 30 or greater. (To calculate your BMI, see page 22.) If you have too much body fat — especially around your waist — you're at greater risk of heart disease and stroke, even if you don't have any other risk factors. Excess weight strains your heart. It also raises your blood pressure and cholesterol levels and increases your chances of developing diabetes. If you're overweight, talk to your doctor about creating a healthy weight-loss plan that's right for you.

• **Diabetes** — If you have diabetes, you're at greater risk of heart disease. Diabetes raises your cholesterol levels. In addition, people with diabetes often have high blood pressure. Type 2 diabetes (non-insulin-dependent diabetes) is the most common type of diabetes and often appears after age 45. Even if your diabetes is under control, you're still at greater risk of heart disease and stroke than a person who doesn't have diabetes. (For information on how you can lower your risk of diabetes, see page 15.)

Risk factors you can't control

• **Age** — Your risk of heart disease increases with age. Four out of five people who die from heart disease are age 65 or older.

• **Sex** — Men are at greater risk of having a heart attack and at an earlier age than women. A woman's risk of a heart attack increases after menopause when estrogen levels decrease.

• **Heredity** — Your risk of heart disease is greater if you have a parent or sibling with heart disease.

• **Race** — Blacks tend to have more severe high blood pressure, which puts them at greater risk of heart disease. Mexican Americans, American Indians, native Hawaiians and Asian Americans are also at greater risk of heart disease. Contributing factors include higher rates of obesity and diabetes — both risk factors for heart disease.

Are you at risk of heart disease?

Check all risk factors that apply to you. Discuss any risk factors with your doctor.

___ I smoke

___ I have high blood pressure

___ I have undesirable cholesterol levels

___ I don't exercise regularly

___ I'm obese

___ I have diabetes

___ I'm age 65 or older

___ I'm male

___ I'm a postmenopausal female

___ I have a family history of heart disease

___ I'm black, Mexican American, American Indian, native Hawaiian or Asian American

Cancer

Cancer is no longer an automatic death sentence. There are many effective treatments for cancer. You can also reduce your risk of getting cancer in the first place. The most common forms of cancer are lung, colon, breast and prostate. The American Cancer Society has identified these risk factors for cancer:

Risk factors you can control

• **Smoking** — In the early 1900s, lung cancer was rare. As cigarettes became mass-produced, the incidence of lung cancer increased dramatically. Smoking is a factor in more than 80 percent of cases of lung cancer. There's also a link between smoking and many other cancers, including those of the pancreas, esophagus, larynx and cervix. (For information on how you can stop smoking, see page 29.)

• **High-fat diet** — According to the American Cancer Society, a high-fat diet increases your risk of many types of cancer. A high-fat diet typically lacks fruits and vegetables — which seem to offer protection against cancer. To reduce your risk of cancer, eat a high-fiber, low-fat diet, including plenty of fruits and vegetables.

• **Excessive alcohol use** — Excessive drinking is linked to several types of cancer, including cancer of the liver, esophagus and breast. Excessive drinking can lead to cirrhosis of the liver — a risk factor for liver cancer. Although the link between alcohol and some other cancers is clear, the cause isn't. Drink alcohol in moderation, if at all. Moderate drinking is defined as no more than two alcoholic beverages a day for men under age 65 and one a day for non-pregnant women and anyone age 65 or older.

• **Exposure to toxins** — Exposure to asbestos and certain chemicals, such as cadmium and some herbicides and pesticides, increases your risk of cancer. Your risk is even greater if you also smoke.

• **Excessive sun exposure** — Overexposure to the sun's ultraviolet radiation can increase your risk of skin cancer. When outdoors, wear sunscreen with an SPF (sun protection factor) of at least 15 and protective clothing such as long sleeves or a broad-brimmed hat.

Risk factors you can't control

• **Family history** — You're at greater risk of cancer if you have a family history of the disease. In some cases, you share a genetic predisposition for the disease. In other cases, you may have been exposed to the same cancer-causing agent, such as cigarette smoke.

• **Age** — Your chances of developing most types of cancer increases after age 50. For this reason, your doctor may recommend more frequent medical exams and cancer screening tests after age 50.

• **Sex** — Some cancers are exclusive to one sex — for example, ovarian and uterine cancers in women, and prostate and testicular cancers in men. Other types of cancers may be more prevalent in men or women. (See chart below.)

• **Race** — Your race may put you at greater risk of certain types of cancer. (See chart below.)

Sex and cancer

Type of cancer	Who's at greater risk?
Lung	Women
Pancreas	Men
Stomach	Men
Esophageal	Men
Kidneys	Men

Race and cancer

Type of cancer	Who's at greater risk?
Breast	Caucasian women get breast cancer more often. However, black women are more likely to die from breast cancer.
Prostate	Black men are twice as likely as Caucasian men to develop prostate cancer.
Esophageal	Blacks are three times more likely than Caucasians to develop esophageal cancer.
Pancreas	Blacks are more likely to develop pancreatic cancer than Caucasians.

• **Personal medical history** — You're at greater risk of cancer if you've had cancer. In addition, other medical conditions can increase your risk of cancer. (See chart below.)

Other conditions and cancer

Medical condition/disease	Increases your risk of
Surgery to remove part of your stomach as treatment for a noncancerous disease, such as obesity or ulcer	Stomach cancer
Hepatitis B and cirrhosis of the liver	Liver cancer
Barrett's esophagus (an inflammation of your esophagus caused by prolonged exposure to stomach acid)	Esophageal cancer
Previous breast cancer in one breast	A new cancer in either breast
Previous cancer in one lung	A new cancer in either lung
Diabetes	Pancreatic cancer

HEALTH RISK ASSESSMENT

Are you at risk of cancer?

Check all risk factors that apply to you. Discuss any risk factors with your doctor.

___ I smoke

___ I eat a high-fat diet

___ I drink alcohol excessively

___ I've been exposed to toxins such as secondhand cigarette smoke, pesticides and herbicides, or asbestos

___ I have a personal or family history of cancer

___ I have a medical condition that puts me at greater risk of cancer

___ My race puts me at higher risk for one or more types of cancer

Lung disease

Chronic obstructive pulmonary disease (COPD) is the overall term for a group of long-standing (chronic) conditions that result in obstruction of your airways. COPD typically refers to two disorders:

• **Chronic bronchitis** — This is a chronic inflammation and thickening of the walls of your bronchial tubes, which narrows them. It often induces coughing spells with excessive amounts of mucus.

• **Emphysema (em-fuh-SEE-muh)** — With emphysema, inflammation damages the walls of your air sacs (alveoli). Your air sacs can lose their natural elasticity, become overstretched and rupture. Small bronchial tubes can collapse and obstruct airflow. Air that you can't exhale before you need to inhale again gets trapped in your lungs and you become short of breath.

You can develop chronic bronchitis and emphysema independently, but most people with COPD have both. Several other lung disorders — chronic bronchial asthma, cystic fibrosis, bronchiolitis and bronchiectasis — are also sometimes classified as COPD because they have similar symptoms and effects.

Risk factors you can control

• **Smoking** — Smoking is the main cause of COPD. You have about a 1 in 4 chance of developing COPD if you smoke. In addition to the irritating effects of smoke on your bronchial tubes, tobacco smoke may damage the cells that preserve normal lung elasticity. Decreased elasticity reduces your ability to exhale oxygen-poor, carbon dioxide-rich air. As a result, your body has trouble maintaining its normal chemical balance, especially during exertion. If you smoke, stop. (For information on how you can quit smoking, see the Stop Smoking Planner on page 29.)

• **Pollutants** — If your occupation exposes you to chemical fumes or dusts from grain, cotton, wood, mining or other sources, you have a higher risk of COPD.

• **Secondhand smoke** — Long-term exposure to secondhand cigarette smoke may increase your risk of COPD if you have other risk factors, such as if you used to smoke.

Risk factors you can't control

• **Heredity** — A less common cause of COPD is an inherited condition known as alpha$_1$-antitrypsin deficiency. A protein in your blood called alpha$_1$-antitrypsin helps protect the air sacs in your lungs from damage due to infection or inflammation. If you're deficient in this protein, you're more likely to develop emphysema at a young age — especially if you smoke. Only about 1 in 2,500 people has this deficiency, which can be detected by a blood test. Although the test is not routinely performed, your doctor may recommend you have the test if you have a family history of COPD, specifically emphysema.

Are you at risk of lung disease?

Check all risk factors that apply to you. Discuss any risk factors with your doctor.

___ I smoke

___ My occupation exposes me to pollutants such as chemical fumes or dust from grain, cotton, wood or mining

___ I've had long-term exposure to secondhand cigarette smoke

___ I have a family history of lung disease

Diabetes

Nearly 6 percent of people in the United States have diabetes. Diabetes is actually a group of diseases with one thing in common — a problem with insulin. The problem could be that your body doesn't make any insulin, doesn't make enough insulin or doesn't use insulin properly.

Insulin is a hormone secreted by your pancreas. It's a key part of the way your body processes the food you eat because it helps maintain the proper level of sugar (glucose) in your blood. Glucose is your body's fuel. Cells use it to produce energy to grow and function. But when you have diabetes, your lack of insulin or the resistance of your cells to insulin prevents the right amount of glucose from entering your cells. The unused glucose builds up in your blood, a condition called hyperglycemia (hi-pur-gli-SEE-me-uh).

There are two types of diabetes:

• Type 1 (insulin dependent)

• Type 2 (non-insulin dependent)

Type 2 is the most common form of diabetes.

Risk factors you can control

• **Overweight** — The more overweight you are, the more resistant your cells become to insulin. Losing weight decreases that resistance. In some cases, just losing weight may bring blood sugar back into normal range. Even a small weight loss may have beneficial effects.

• **Sedentary lifestyle** — Regular exercise helps you control your weight. In addition, your body uses more glucose during exercise, which helps lower your glucose levels.

Risk factors you can't control

• **Age** — You're at greater risk of type 2 diabetes after age 45. As a result, your doctor may recommend more frequent screening tests for diabetes.

• **Family history** — You have a greater chance of developing type 2 diabetes if a grandparent, parent or sibling has it.

• **Race** — You're at greater risk of type 2 diabetes if you're black, Hispanic or American Indian.

• **Pregnancy-related diabetes** —You're at greater risk of type 2 diabetes if you've had pregnancy-related (gestational) diabetes.

HEALTH RISK ASSESSMENT

Are you at risk of diabetes?

Check all risk factors that apply to you. Discuss any risk factors with your doctor.

__ I'm overweight

__ I don't exercise regularly

__ I'm older than 45

__ I have a family history of diabetes

__ My race puts me at greater risk of diabetes

__ I've had pregnancy-related diabetes

Kidney disease

Many different diseases or events can damage your kidneys and cause them to fail. It can happen suddenly or take place gradually over months or years. Common conditions include diabetes, high blood pressure and an inflammation of the kidneys called glomerulonephritis (glo-mer-u-lo-nuh-FRI-tis). Inherited kidney diseases, the most common of which is polycystic kidney disease, can also cause kidney failure.

When your kidneys aren't able to function at more than 10 percent of normal capacity, you need kidney dialysis (an artificial way to remove your body's waste and extra fluid) or a kidney transplant to survive. This condition is known as end-stage renal (kidney) disease.

Risk factors you can control

• **Diabetes and high blood pressure** — Diabetes and high blood pressure are the two most common diseases that damage your kidneys. High blood pressure stresses the walls of your blood vessels. If the blood vessels in your kidneys are damaged, they may not remove wastes from your blood as efficiently. This increases your blood pressure even more. Diabetes slowly damages your kidneys. It's not understood how diabetes causes kidney disease. However, research shows if you have high blood pressure and diabetes, you're at greater risk of developing kidney disease. Managing these diseases is key to preventing kidney disease. Note: One group of high blood pressure medications, called ACE inhibitors, helps protect your kidneys, especially if you also have diabetes.

Risk factors you can't control

• **Heredity** — At least three types of kidney disease are hereditary. These include lupus nephritis (caused by a disease of the immune system), hereditary nephritis and polycystic renal disease.

HEALTH RISK ASSESSMENT

Are you at risk of kidney disease?

Check all risk factors that apply to you. Discuss any risk factors with your doctor.

___ I have diabetes or high blood pressure, which puts me at higher risk of kidney disease

___ I have a family history of kidney disease

Take charge of your health

What are your health risk "trouble spots" — lifestyle activities or habits that increase your risk of disease? Do you smoke? Do you drink alcohol excessively? Are you physically inactive? Eat poorly?

The good news is you can change risky lifestyle habits. Identify where you need to improve. Then make a plan for change. You're more likely to succeed if you don't try to tackle everything at once. To start, target one or two areas. Then gradually add more goals, one at a time.

Change can be difficult. However, when you understand how risky behaviors can hurt your health, you may find more strength to adopt healthier habits. Here's what we know about five risky lifestyle habits.

Smoking

Smoking causes lung cancer, lung disease, heart disease and stroke. It also aggravates other chronic illnesses, such as diabetes and asthma. Smoking is the cause of more premature deaths than any other lifestyle habit.

Fortunately, as soon as you stop smoking, your risk of heart disease and stroke drops dramatically. Ten years after you quit, your risk of stroke is about the same as that of a nonsmoker. Even if you quit after age 60, you may add 5 to 7 years to your life.

Why is smoking so bad for you?

• Smoking damages the walls of your blood vessels, making them prone to buildup of cholesterol-containing fatty deposits called plaque (atherosclerosis).

• Smoking may also reduce the proportion of HDL (or "good") cholesterol to LDL (or "bad") cholesterol in your blood. High levels of LDL cholesterol increase your risk of atherosclerosis.

By contrast, high HDL levels are protective because they may prevent formation of plaque.

• Smoking is responsible for 85 percent or more of all lung cancers. An aggressive kind — small cell carcinoma — is found almost exclusively in smokers.

• Carbon monoxide in cigarette smoke replaces oxygen in your blood. This also increases blood pressure by forcing your heart to work harder to supply adequate oxygen.

Chewing tobacco can also be harmful — causing cancer of the mouth, tongue and throat.

If you use tobacco, stop. To learn more about stop-smoking methods, see page 29.

Drinking alcohol excessively

Excessive drinking can raise your blood pressure and damage your organs, especially your liver. Heavy drinking also increases your risk of death from all causes including cancer and stroke.

Drink alcohol in moderation, if at all. Moderate drinking is defined as no more than one alcoholic drink a day for nonpregnant women and anyone age 65 or older and two a day for men under 65. One drink is 12 ounces of regular beer, 5 ounces of wine or 1.5 ounces of 80-proof distilled spirits.

Sedentary lifestyle

A sedentary lifestyle puts you at risk for becoming overweight, which is a risk factor for several diseases. (To find out if you're overweight, see "Calculate your body mass index" on page 22.) Regular exercise can:

• Help prevent coronary artery disease and stroke

• Help reduce high blood pressure

• Help prevent and control type 2 diabetes

• Prevent bone loss and osteoporosis

• Help control weight and prevent obesity when combined with a healthy diet

Find a physical activity you like, and stick with it. Aim for 3 to 4 hours a week (about 30 minutes per day) of moderately intense activity. This includes brisk walking, swimming and biking. If you're older than age 50 or have a chronic health problem, talk to your doctor before starting a vigorous exercise program.

To learn more about how to start an exercise program, see the Exercise Planner on page 26.

Eating an unhealthy diet

A high-fat diet increases your risk of many types of cancer. It also puts you at risk of obesity — a risk factor for many diseases, including heart disease and diabetes. (To find out if you're overweight, see "Calculate your body mass index" on page 22.)

Eating a low-fat diet rich in grains, fruits and vegetables can help prevent diseases. It also helps you maintain a healthy weight. Here are some dietary guidelines:

• **Fruits and vegetables** — Eat 5 to 9 servings a day. Eating plenty of fruits and vegetables is the best way to get antioxidants — chemicals that help prevent buildup of cholesterol-containing fatty deposits called plaque (atherosclerosis) in your blood vessels. Fruits and vegetables also contain soluble fiber that may help lower cholesterol.

• **Meat, fish and poultry** — Eat 2 or fewer servings a day. Choose lean meat and skinless poultry to reduce the amount of fat you get. Fish contains a type of polyunsaturated fat called omega-3 fatty acids, which may protect against coronary artery disease. These fats can help improve cholesterol levels and may help lower blood pressure slightly. Omega-3 fatty acids occur naturally in cold-water fish such as salmon and mackerel.

• **Dairy products** — Eat 2 to 3 servings a day. Dairy products are key sources of calcium and vitamin D, which helps your body absorb calcium. They also provide protein. But, dairy products can be high in fat. By choosing low-fat or fat-free varieties, such as skim or low-fat milk and yogurt, and fat-free or part-skim cheeses, you can get the health benefits of dairy products without all the fat.

• **Grains** — Eat 6 to 11 servings a day. Grains include breads, cereals, rice and pasta. In addition to being low in fat, grains are rich in complex carbohydrates and nutrients. They're also a good source of insoluble fiber, found mainly in whole grains. This kind of fiber helps prevent constipation and may possibly reduce your risk of colon cancer.

To learn how to improve your diet, see the Nutrition Planner on page 23.

Obesity

You're obese if your body mass index (BMI) is 30 or greater. (To calculate your BMI, see page 22.) Being overweight makes you more likely to have high blood pressure or heart disease. It also increases your resistance to insulin and is the leading cause of type 2 diabetes (non-insulin-dependent diabetes). When you're overweight or obese, your liver makes more triglycerides and cholesterol, making you more vulnerable to heart disease. You're also at increased risk of developing gallstones and cancer of the breast, prostate, colon and uterus.

In addition, if you're even moderately overweight, you're carrying a constant burden on your back and legs. Eventually, this can aggravate conditions such as degenerative arthritis (osteoarthritis).

To learn how you can achieve and maintain a healthy weight, see the Nutrition Planner on page 21 and the Exercise Planner on page 26.

A successful program to make any lifestyle changes requires that you set specific, attainable goals. Use the planners on the following pages to help you get started on your way to better health.

Calculate your body mass index (BMI)

To calculate your BMI, find your height in the left-hand column. Then find your weight in the row to the right of your height. When you find it, the number at the top of that column is your BMI. If your BMI falls between 18.5 and 24.9, you're at a healthy weight. If your BMI is 25 or over, you're overweight. If your BMI is 30 or greater, you're obese. Asians with a BMI over 23 may have an increased risk of health problems.

Body mass index (BMI)

	HEALTHY		OVERWEIGHT					OBESE				
BMI	19	24	25	26	27	28	29	30	35	40	45	50
HEIGHT			**WEIGHT IN POUNDS**									
4'10"	91	115	119	124	129	134	138	143	167	191	215	239
4'11"	94	119	124	128	133	138	143	148	173	198	222	247
5'0"	97	123	128	133	138	143	148	153	179	204	230	255
5'1"	100	127	132	137	143	148	153	158	185	211	238	264
5'2"	104	131	136	142	147	153	158	164	191	218	246	273
5'3"	107	135	141	146	152	158	163	169	197	225	254	282
5'4"	110	140	145	151	157	163	169	174	204	232	262	291
5'5"	114	144	150	156	162	168	174	180	210	240	270	300
5'6"	118	148	155	161	167	173	179	186	216	247	278	309
5'7"	121	153	159	166	172	178	185	191	223	255	287	319
5'8"	125	158	164	171	177	184	190	197	230	262	295	328
5'9"	128	162	169	176	182	189	196	203	236	270	304	338
5'10"	132	167	174	181	188	195	202	209	243	278	313	348
5'11"	136	172	179	186	193	200	208	215	250	286	322	358
6'0"	140	177	184	191	199	206	213	221	258	294	331	368
6'1"	144	182	189	197	204	212	219	227	265	302	340	378
6'2"	148	186	194	202	210	218	225	233	272	311	350	389
6'3"	152	192	200	208	216	224	232	240	279	319	359	399
6'4"	156	197	205	213	221	230	238	246	287	328	369	410

Modified from National Institutes of Health Clinical Guidelines on the Identification, Evaluation, and Treatment of Overweight and Obesity in Adults, 1998.

Nutrition Planner

MAINTAIN GOOD NUTRITION

The simplest way to maintain good nutrition is to follow the dietary recommendation of the Food Guide Pyramid. Start by following at least one of the recommendations below. Work up to following all six.

____ I eat 6 to 11 servings of bread, cereal, rice or pasta each day.

____ I eat 3 to 5 servings of vegetables each day.

____ I eat 2 to 4 servings of fruit each day.

____ I eat no more than 2 to 3 servings of meat, poultry, eggs, or nuts each day.

____ I eat or drink 2 servings of milk or dairy products each day.

____ I limit the amount of fats, oils and sweets I eat each day.

SET YOUR GOALS

The easiest way to make permanent changes in how you eat is to take small steps. The following tool can help you establish weekly goals and rewards. Under each category select one weekly goal — more if you're game. Don't forget to treat yourself to something special when you achieve your goals. Set new goals each week when the previous ones are met and maintained. The options listed below are to get you started. Make up your own and write them down.

The five food groups *Select 1*

____ I will eat a piece of fruit with dinner.

____ I will eat one vegetable with dinner.

____ I will not eat fried food with dinner.

____ Your own goal: _____

Cooking right *Select 1*

____ I will experiment with a food I've never tried before.

____ I will prepare a meal with a variety of food colors and textures.

____ I will prepare a meatless dinner.

____ Your own goal: _____

Nutrition Planner

Good eating habits *Select 1*

___ I will have juice with cereal or toast for breakfast.

___ I will have a fresh green salad with my restaurant order.

___ I will snack on apples and carrot sticks.

___ Your own goal: _____

Smart food choices *Select 1*

___ I will compare the sodium or sugar content on food labels of products.

___ I will prepare a shopping list before I go to the grocery store.

___ I will not shop for food when I'm hungry.

___ Your own goal: _____

Social support *Select 1*

___ I will call a friend when I'm tempted to snack more than I should.

___ I will share a vegetable or fruit snack with a friend.

___ I will sit down to dinner with my family or friends.

___ Your own goal: _____

Reward *Select 1*

___ I will plan to call or meet with a friend I haven't contacted in a while.

___ I will take time to pursue a favorite hobby.

___ I will go to a movie, concert or play.

___ Your own reward: _____

SHOP WISELY

How well you carry out your nutrition plan depends a great deal on what you have on hand to eat. Here are some savvy shopping strategies to help you stock your kitchen with healthy foods and ingredients.

• **Plan ahead.** Before you go shopping, decide how many major meals you're going to buy for on this shopping trip. Then, think through the

Nutrition Planner

number of other food items you'll need for breakfasts, lunches and snacks in that time period. Take an inventory of your staples.

• **Make a shopping list.** A list will make your shopping trip more efficient and help you avoid impulse purchases. If you generally shop in the same store, write a master list, with items you normally buy in the order that you travel through the store. Make copies to use during each shopping adventure, just adding items specifically for the recipes you plan to make.

• **Add an indulgence to the list.** Perhaps one favorite dessert, a food with a short season or a new convenience item. Don't let a previous list prevent you from looking for and trying new foods.

• **Don't shop when you're hungry.** It's harder to resist quick snacks when you need something to eat. These packaged foods are often high in calories, fat and sodium. If you do find yourself shopping on an empty stomach, drink some water or buy a piece of fruit to munch on while you shop.

• **Be an informed shopper.** Talk to store personnel for advice on the best quality available. For packaged goods, learn the packaging terminology and read the food labels. If you don't always have time, choose one item in each shopping trip. For example, read the labels of ready-to-eat cereals, looking for whole grains in the ingredient lists and comparing fiber amounts among brands. Soon you'll know the foods to buy without spending time reading the labels all the time.

Exercise Planner

GET STARTED

Talk to your physician before you start a new exercise program if you're a woman older than 50, a man older than 40, or have a chronic health problem, such as arthritis, asthma or high blood pressure.

DESIGN YOUR PROGRAM

Fitness generally includes four components — aerobic capacity, strength, flexibility and weight control. This last component may be achieved by your exercise program and sensible eating.

When you design your program, keep these points in mind:

• **Make a plan.** A written plan will encourage you to stay on track, and a diary or log will help you chart your progress.

• **Plan a logical progression.** If you have unstable joints from injury or arthritis, or you're in a weakened condition, start by improving your muscle strength and flexibility first. Build strength using light weights, exercising the weakest parts of your body.

• **Start at a comfortable level.** Try walking 5 to 10 minutes over a short distance indoors. Increase 1 to 5 minutes per session, as tolerated.

• **Schedule regular exercise.** For your fitness to improve, you need to exercise regularly. Aim for 3 to 4 hours a week (about 30 minutes a day) of low- to moderate-intensity physical activity.

• **Include variety.** Combine three types of exercise — stretching (flexibility), endurance (aerobic) and strengthening (weight training) — and three levels of intensity — warm-up, workout level and cooldown — in each exercise session.

• **Cross-training reduces your risk of injury.** Alternate among exercises that emphasize different parts of the body, such as swimming, bicycling and walking.

• **Don't overdo.** Many people start with frenzied zeal — exercising too long or too intensely — and give up when muscles and joints become sore or injured. Start slowly and build up gradually, allowing time between sessions for your body to rest and recover. If pain occurs repeatedly in your muscles or joints during exercise, cut back and seek guidance from your doctor.

Exercise Planner

SET YOUR GOALS

Use this weekly goal-setting tool to help you stick with your exercise plan as you work to improve your overall fitness. In most cases, the options are suggestions to help you set specific goals each week.

Warm-up/Cool-down

___ I will do proper stretching before and after exercising.

Exercise *Select 1 or 2*

___ Aerobic dancing

___ Bicycling

___ Dancing

___ Gardening

___ Golf (carry or pull your bag — no carts!)

___ Swimming

___ Walking (30 minutes)

___ Your own goal: _____

Strength exercises *Select 1*

___ I will do strength training once this week.

___ I will do strength training twice this week.

___ I will do strength training three times this week.

___ Your own goal: _____

Other activities *Select 1 or 2*

___ I will clean the house.

___ I will garden.

___ I will mow the lawn.

___ Your own goal: _____

Exercise Planner

Social support *Select 1*

___ I will ask my family for encouragement.

___ I will exercise with a friend or family member.

___ I will review my progress with my family or friend.

___ Your own goal: _____

Reward *Select 1*

___ I will get a massage.

___ I will go fishing or camping.

___ I will visit a museum.

___ Your own goal: _____

Stop Smoking Planner

CREATE A PLAN

Becoming smoke-free is a result of planning and commitment, not luck. The best results combine medication with some form of structured assistance to help you change your smoking behavior — group support or individual counseling, for instance.

Your "stop plan" should combine various strategies, or plans of action, for:

- Coping with symptoms of nicotine withdrawal
- Resisting urges to smoke
- Improving overall physical and emotional health
- Gaining social support and guidance, when necessary

No one plan works for everybody — in the same way there is no one right way to stop smoking. Build a stop plan that you are most likely to follow. Choose various techniques and tools that you feel suit your needs. These choices become your "strategies" to stop smoking.

There are several strategies to help you stop smoking. Review each one and then choose what strategies you will use and how.

Self-help — Work with available health resources to plan and maintain your stop smoking plan. Resources include the American Cancer Society, American Lung Association and Centers for Disease Control, as well as state and local public health departments. You can also find a stop smoking planner on the Mayo Clinic Web site at www.MayoClinic.com.

Group support — Meet with other individuals working to become smoke-free. Led by a trained group leader, you meet regularly in an organized smoking cessation program. For information on stop smoking clinics or groups, contact the American Cancer Society, American Lung Association or local public health department. Some businesses maintain smoking cessation clinics for their employees.

Individual counseling — Arrange for one-on-one contact with a trusted doctor, psychologist, nurse or counselor. Trained professionals allow you to express your feelings, your fears of not being able to stop, or problems with family or friends. They help you gain coping skills, overcome obstacles and learn to live as a nonsmoker.

Cold turkey — This is a sudden decisive break from cigarettes. On a chosen day, you stop smoking completely with little or no reduction

Stop Smoking Planner

beforehand. Going cold turkey requires preparation to withstand the strong symptoms of nicotine withdrawal. Doctors usually recommend some form of medication for moderate to heavy smokers who want to use this method.

Medication — Doctors may recommend medication for heavy smokers. Medication helps reduce your craving for cigarettes and eases the withdrawal symptoms of nicotine. There are two basic types of medication. FDA-approved nicotine replacement products — such as patches, gum or nasal spray — deliver safer, controlled amounts of nicotine to your brain via your bloodstream — without smoking. A non-nicotine antidepressant, bupropion (Zyban), is also available to help people stop smoking. Bupropion is also marketed under the name Wellbutrin for the treatment of depression. Don't use more than one form of bupropion at a time. In addition, don't use bupropion if you've recently taken a monoamine oxidase inhibitor (MAOI) or if you have a history of seizures, head trauma, stroke, anorexia or bulimia. If you have high blood pressure, heart disease, kidney or liver disease, or you regularly drink alcohol or take benzodiazepines (Valium, Librium, Xanax, others), ask your doctor about the risks of using bupropion.

Alternative therapies — Hypnosis or acupuncture may help relieve nicotine withdrawal. However, these treatments aren't in themselves effective long-term strategies to stop smoking.

Strategy	*What I will do*
Self-help	____ Read printed material from health organizations
	____ Do research on nicotine addiction and how to stop smoking
	Your own ideas: _____
Group support	____ Find a "stopping" buddy — a nonsmoking friend or family member — to help me through tough times and moments to celebrate my success
	____ Call a local health organization about support groups
	____ Enroll in a stop smoking program
	____ Your own ideas: _____

Stop Smoking Planner

Individual counseling	___	Contact a health professional with questions and concerns
	___	Have ongoing counseling sessions with a professional
	___	Your ideas: _____
Other methods	___	Talk to my doctor about medication to help ease the withdrawal symptoms of nicotine
	___	Check out alternative therapies such as hypnosis or acupuncture
	___	Start exercising
	___	Your own ideas: _____

CHOOSE A STOP DAY

You have your strategies in place. Now it's time to decide when to put the cigarettes away.

The day you set as your personal stop day should be *within two weeks* of the moment you make the decision to stop smoking. That's when your motivation is high. Make a real effort to stick to this day.

Most people choose to stop smoking during a relatively low-stress time in their lives. Sometimes those periods are difficult to find — but don't let that stop you.

Consider the factors listed below as you choose your stop day. Some of them may be important to you, while others may not. You decide what would work best for you:

• A day of low stress

• A day away from the office, such as on weekends or vacations

• A day when you aren't involved in your everyday routine

• An open day that fits easily within your work and personal schedules

• A busy day that keeps your mind and hands occupied

• A day when family and friends you depend on aren't under stress

Becoming smoke-free requires commitment. Believe that you can be successful. Prepare to deal with periods of stress or depression. Remember your reasons for wanting to be smoke-free. Doing this can increase your motivation and confidence.

Healthy living — One step at a time

Reviewing your health habits, then making a plan for change and carrying it out may seem like a daunting task. But if you proceed one step at a time, living a healthy lifestyle will become an attainable goal.

Each step complements and builds on the next, increasing your momentum. Eating less fat leads to eating more fruits and vegetables. Eating a healthy diet helps you lose weight. Losing weight makes it easier to exercise and so on. Each of these changes also helps improve your view of yourself, further motivating you to continue to work toward better health.

A healthy lifestyle may not be enough to prevent you from developing disease. You also may need medication and other medical intervention. However, your lifestyle is the one area you can control. And whether it helps prevent disease or improves treatment of an illness you already have, a healthy lifestyle is a critical factor in the quality of your life.

GLOSSARY

Alveoli: Small air sacs in the lungs.

Body mass index (BMI): A measurement that relates your body weight to health risks associated with being overweight.

Cadmium: A chemical used in the manufacture of certain products, such as rechargeable batteries. Exposure to this chemical increases your risk of cancer.

Chronic obstructive pulmonary disease (COPD): The term for a group of long-standing (chronic) conditions that result in obstruction of your airways. Examples are emphysema and chronic bronchitis.

Glomerulonephritis: An inflammation of the kidneys.

Insulin: A hormone secreted by the pancreas that is essential for the metabolism of carbohydrates and the body's maintenance of a sugar (glucose). A lack of or resistance in the cells to insulin can result in diabetes.

Polycystic kidney disease: With this condition, the kidneys contain clusters of cysts that interfere with function and enlarge the kidneys.

Risk factor: Anything that makes you susceptible to developing a disease.

INDEX

Blood pressure, 6-7
Body mass index, 21-22

Cholesterol, 6

Diet, 20-21, 23-25

Exercise, 19-20, 26-28

Health risk assessment
    cancer, 12
    diabetes, 16
    heart disease, 9
    kidney disease, 17
    lung disease, 14

Smoking cessation, 18, 29-31